My Conceptual Self-Conception Journal/Workbook

Have you ever wondered why you believe some or all of the things that you do? Or are most of the things that you believe about yourself really true? Do you ever question some of the decisions that you make? Or wonder why you seem to make the same mistakes, over & over again? Have you ever wondered why certain things just seem to happen to you? Or do you constantly feel like you're around people that always seem to annoy you?

Well your self-concept, or the things that you believe about yourself plays a major part in how you react to certain situations and in how certain people react towards you and how they ultimately see you in life.

The concept that you have about yourself at this moment has been shaped by your past. Or rather, your perception of your past. By reviewing the uncomfortable experiences from your past, you will be able to change your thoughts surrounding them and then find, a more positive resolution. Remember that the past is over and it is no indication of what the future will hold. The past is only a limitation if you allow it to be.

With this workbook you will discover ways to form a healthy concept about yourself, examine your past to see if there are any negative or inaccurate beliefs that need to be adjusted and then create ways to empower your self-esteem and build your self-worth.

So the first task on your agenda is to ask yourself, Who am I? Who do you see yourself as? What type of person do you believe you are? Are you strong? Are you confident? Are you smart? What is, your concept of you? And most importantly where did this concept originate from?

Because it may be possible that, a lot of the things that you believe about yourself may not be true or entirely accurate.

We all have a history, filled with negative and positive experiences that we begin to interpret and assign labels to, then these experiences leave an impression on us and that is how we will see them & judge them in the future.

Now, there are certain things about ourselves that we can not change. Like our race, our parents, etc. But there are a lot of things that we can change, if we don't like the results we're seeing in our lives. As stated, our past experiences, form our future decisions, and there are several signs that will prove if those experiences are having a negative or positive effect on your life. Let's look at a few:

- You consistently make the same mistakes in life - by examining your past, you should be able to discern why you make the same mistakes over & over if you take the time to accurately dissect the experience
- You adopt the attitude(s), beliefs or behavioral characteristics of your parent(s) - what worked for your parents may not necessarily work for you, you don't know what caused them to believe what they believe. Any belief that you haven't formed based on the current situation and the facts surrounding it, can be dangerous and further more damaging to your self-image.

- You flat out ignore your past - Although this is sometimes the easiest thing to do, especially if there is a lot of pain and hardship involved, but the consequences or fruit so to speak, will still be there and evident throughout your life as long as you continue to neglect the responsibility of dealing with it. It will be like weeds, choking out the true you and stifling your self-image and concept.
- Any traumatic experience from your childhood - this could be anything from a situation that you were involved in(you were injured, heart broken, or teased in school), or something that you witnessed (an accident, a t.v. show, a fight), or something that happened to your family (a death, divorce, etc.)

One bad thought or belief for that matter can affect your whole life if left unanalyzed & processed accurately. We have to constantly challenge our beliefs, especially when we find ourselves producing unwanted fruit or negative results consistently. But sometimes it's hard to recognize our own flaws, especially when we don't have any honest feedback or people that we respect and trust in our lives.

So let's look at a few ways to determine if your past is negatively affecting you:

1. Make a list of the things that you believe about yourself. Try to focus on negative beliefs and limitations only. Include every area where you feel neglected or dissatisfied.

For Example:
- I can't lose weight
- I'll never get married
- I'm always late
- I'll never have a good job
- All men/women are cheaters/liars

2. Question each belief. Many of our beliefs are not completely justified, if we take the time to examine them, we can run them through a quick filter of questions to see if they are worth holding on to.

- Where or from Whom did this belief originate?
- Is it based on truth or a similar experience? Placing our hands into fire is a truth that fire will burn, eating one or even two bad apples, is not sufficient enough truth, to say that all apples are bad.
- Is the belief rational?

3. What is this belief costing you? False beliefs can cost and cause a lot of damages in your life. Measure the cost of the things that you believe, they can produce:

- Unhealthy relationships
- A lack of confidence
- A lower income
- Overall dissatisfaction in life itself
- Stagnation in every major area

4. Choose another belief. Find a belief that supports the person that you truly are, or choose to be. One that supports the life you desire to have. Turn I can't lose weight into, By feeding my body the proper nutrients, and beginning to burn the excess energy that I'm currently storing, I will lose weight, because all extra weight is, is extra energy that I haven't used.

5. Find evidence to support your new belief. Because your mind will continue to dwell on the past. The past failures and attempts, and without evidence to support your new belief, it will be hard to convince your inner self that the new belief is possible or true.

It's not uncommon, to be limited by our past. Because we are for the most part creatures of habit. But what we fail to realize is that, all behavior is learned. We didn't come into this world knowing anything, & at some point we had to learn everything that we now know and believe, but the fact is, Not all of it is accurate and Not all of it is based on truth or reality. So as we mature, some of the things that we believe must also mature, and be analyzed. Like at one point you may have believed in everything from the boogieman to Santa, the easter bunny and the tooth fairy, but once you became a teenager hopefully those beliefs changed. In the same way, as you continue to mature the things you believed as a teenager should change, and you should continue to evaluate and reevaluate your beliefs for the rest of your life.

So here's a little homework to get you started:

- Make a new list of all of your negative beliefs about yourself. Then focus on one belief at a time
- Question the belief
- Determine exactly what the belief is costing you
- Choose an alternative belief
- Then find evidence to support your new belief
- Then move to another until you have went through your whole list

Puzzle #1
I AM PUZZLE

```
Z E V I T A E R C L A Y O L Q
M M N G D N X O B A T B O D P
E L G E N E A G P D T C L P A
N L T X V I C I L E E A S E S
T J B T D I V I L D N F X A S
H A T I N E T R S L T X H C I
U L T N X E N A E I I U U E O
S T U T E E D I I S V R M F N
I R K F R C L I M C E E B U A
A U M J E A O F F R E D L L T
S S E A R P C N J N E R E A E
T T U S D M O T N T O T P G D
I I A X I F H H I I P C E P F
C N G V Q W C L E V E R R D A
S G V N C O U R A G E O U S L
```

ABLE   CREATIVE   INNOCENT
APPRECIATIVE   DECISIVE   LOYAL
ATTENTIVE   DESERVING   OPEN
ATTRACTIVE   DETERMINED   PASSIONATE
BRILLIANT   ENTHUSIASTIC   PEACEFUL
CLEVER   FLEXIBLE   TRUSTING
CONFIDENT   HOPEFUL   WISE
COURAGEOUS   HUMBLE

Self-Concept Quiz #1

Choose the correct answer.

1. Is it possible that some of the things you believe about yourself aren't true at all?

    a. Yes
    b. No

2. What is the most relevant item to your self-concept?

    a. The truth about the experiences of your past
    b. What TV shows you watched as a kid
    c. Your dreams when you're asleep
    d. How you interpret the experiences of your past

3. Ignoring your past is the most constructive way to use it.

    a. True
    b. False

4. It's easier to present yourself authentically to others when you can:

    a. Feel good about yourself
    b. Hide your past
    c. Eat as much as you want
    d. All of the above

5. Which strategies will build your self-esteem?

    a. Show off your strengths
    b. Do something for others
    c. Learn something new
    d. All of the above

Puzzle #2

I COULD BE

```
Z  L  U  N  J  O  U  R  N  A  L  I  S  T  B
P  H  Y  S  I  C  I  A  N  U  L  J  W  O  P
R  J  U  D  G  E  I  R  Z  G  R  D  B  R  M
N  E  D  C  R  S  T  H  E  N  J  S  J  T  Y
U  A  T  S  P  O  L  E  O  E  I  D  E  H  S
T  V  I  H  T  T  S  Y  L  A  N  A  S  O  L
R  O  T  C  G  C  N  S  C  H  K  I  G  D  A
I  N  L  U  I  I  E  A  E  R  T  O  G  O  W
T  Q  O  I  A  R  F  T  T  F  J  A  G  N  Y
I  M  A  E  P  N  T  E  I  N  O  E  F  T  E
O  A  H  P  G  O  O  C  R  H  U  R  K  I  R
N  Y  E  R  G  R  Z  R  E  I  C  O  P  S  R
I  O  L  M  P  K  U  D  T  L  F  R  C  T  D
S  R  K  Y  S  A  W  S  G  S  E  V  A  C  U
T  W  D  T  S  I  C  A  M  R  A  H  P  Y  A
```

ACCOUNTANT
ANALYST
ARCHITECT
ASTRONAUT
ATHLETE
ELECTRICIAN
ENGINEER
FIRE FIGHTER

JOURNALIST
JUDGE
LAWYER
MAYOR
NURSE
NUTRITIONIST
ORTHODONTIST
PHARMACIST

PHYSICIAN
PILOT
PROFESSOR
SURGEON

Self-Concept Quiz #2

1. Which situation is more likely to inspire you to change your life?

    a. When you think more highly of yourself
    b. When you think you're a failure, so you should change
    c. Watching an entertaining TV show
    d. All of the above

2. One of the more reliable ways to enhance your self-concept is to:

    a. Watch TV
    b. Make some positive changes
    c. Take a nap
    d. Cheat at a contest to ensure that you'll be the winner

3. Exercising regularly can raise your self-concept.

    a. True
    b. False

4. Setting goals within this timeline is usually the most effective for maintaining focus and enthusiasm:

    a. 10 years
    b. 1 year
    c. 6 months
    d. 12 weeks

5. If you have a healthy self-concept, you shouldn't aspire for more than you have.

    a. True
    b. False

Now as stated before, and as you have probably realized after completing your first assignment when we revisit the past, we can uncover memories or feelings that we have tried to forget. Situations from our childhood or young adulthood, that may have scarred us or held us bound to a negative belief. It's like reopening an old wound and reliving the situation all over again. But at times that is actually what we need to do, especially if we never actually healed or recovered from that situation. We all need to face our demons, so to speak, we need to confront whatever it is that is holding us back. Sometimes there may be people that we need to forgive in order to move forward. There may be old wounds or scars that you need to heal from.

One highly productive and easy strategy to use to uncover and release yourself from past situations is journaling aka writing down how you feel and what you think. Let's explore a few journaling techniques.

Expressing yourself with pen and paper, or even on a computer, will help you discharge your troublesome feelings and move on with your goals. Enjoy your best life now by using journaling to help heal old wounds.

Try these journaling techniques to help you resolve the pain of negative childhood memories:

1. Writing about what you thought and felt. Let's go back in time, pick a rememberable event and ponder about what the negative situation was like for you. Did you feel embarrassed the first time your father missed your parents day meeting at school? Were you angry about Mom's consistent efforts to make you sing in the choir? Write it down.

2. What are your current thoughts and feelings? Next, use your current "adult mind" to take a look at the situation the best you can. What does your adult mind tell you about what really happened? Maybe you see things more clearly now. Was your parents goal to simply make you a "better person?" Jot down your current interpretation of the situation.

3. Document how the challenging situations affected you then. How did you react as a child to what happened? How did you make sense of the trying situations then? Did your Dad miss events because he was busy trying to support the family? Who, if anyone, did you talk to about the troublesome times? Mention them in your journal.

4. Ponder how the hurtful events from the past affect you now. See if you can make any connections between your past and present. Make a conscious decision to better manage your feelings and behavioral choices now. Write down how you can manage your emotions differently.

5. Vow to gain understanding. If it was a situation when your parent did something that you just couldn't understand, can you make sense of it now? Maybe your father didn't make you stay home from a trip to punish you - perhaps he thought you'd be exposed to something unsavory or even unsafe and he was hoping to protect you.

* Explore these possible explanations through writing in your journal.

6. Re-write your history. Re-construct your childhood on paper how you would have liked it to be. It's a learning experience to formulate how you would have liked your growing up years to have been different. Re-writing your history can also help you heal.

7. Make a conscious decision to overcome your past. Whatever your old hurts, decide to disconnect them from your current life. This effort must be made consciously and with great thought. Write down how you can release yourself.

8. Recognize these events were in the past. As you record your thoughts and feelings, make note of how long ago the situation or events occurred. Label them as "in the past" in your journal. Start a new section called, "In the present" and write about how you'll respond to those types of hurts now.

9. Formulate a plan to let it go and move on. In your writings, consider steps you might take to move on in your life and live more openly and without being tethered to your historic pain.

10. Give yourself permission to release the old, negative emotions. In your journal, jot down that you no longer have to carry the hurt. Allow yourself permission to leave it behind you. You can even draw a picture of the tangled web of feelings and state you're leaving all the pain right there between the lines of your journal.

Next we will look at some self forgiveness techniques!

Self forgiveness starts with loving yourself. Forgiving others is another major part of self forgiveness. Sometimes holding grudges and harboring un-forgiveness in your heart leads to bitterness and eventually depression. If you want to forgive yourself, you have to let go of, all of the negative emotions and all past encounters, it's not to say you have to apologize to people who hurt you, but forgiving them helps you heal.

Once you have cleared your conscious of all past hurts and negative attitudes, you can begin to start planting positive seeds in your life, to eliminate the old negative thoughts.

One way to that is through affirmations.

Affirmations help us to keep a positive attitude about life. Writing our own affirmations makes them personal to us, which can then help us to get through our own individual situations. It's only natural that we'll get more out of these positive sayings if we formulate them ourselves. But first, we will start with some pre-written affirmations to help you get on the right track and to begin your healing process. But I suggest getting into the habit of writing out your own affirmations, so that they will be addressing your specific needs and be more effective.

Let's start with letting go of the past hurts, disappointments and negative memories. Repeat these affirmations as often as possible, and try memorizing a few to repeat to yourself when needed.

I release the past.

I feel liberated when I release the past. I let go of the memories that hold me back, and put the past to rest.

I forgive all of those who may have harmed me. I try to understand their position and wish them well, even if I disagree with their actions.

I come to terms with loss. Life is full of transitions. I will make the most of my experiences and relationships while they last. I am comfortable with beginnings and endings.

I learn from my missteps. I forgive myself and move on. Taking sensible risks may sometimes expose me to errors. However, pursuing valuable opportunities is more satisfying than refusing to try at all.

I put the past behind me, I am now able to face my feelings. I examine my thoughts to see if they serve my current interests. I am open to changing my viewpoint.

I live in the present moment. I slow down and pay attention to my senses. I ask myself if I am seeing a situation realistically or whether my vision is distorted by previous experiences.

While I focus on the here and now, I am also planning for the future. I devote my energy to creating positive change and I am hopeful about what lies ahead.

Today, I release myself from the past, I embrace the future and welcome new adventures.

I am free of the challenges of my past.

I choose to leave the past in the past. I am focused on my present and future self. I will remember happy times from my past. But I choose to leave my past challenges behind me where they belong.

I learn from the challenges of the past and then I release them. The past can only exist in my mind if I allow it. I have better uses for my mind than remembering negative events from the past.

The present is my primary focus. I use the present to create my future. I am committed to enjoying every moment as it is happening.

Life can only be lived in the present.

The past is only a mirage of who I used to be. I am constantly growing and evolving. I renew myself each day.

The past is only a snapshot of a time gone by. I learn from the past and then immediately move on. I am grateful for my past challenges since I learn so much from them. After gaining that knowledge, I release my awareness of those challenges.

Each day, I remember to focus on the things that are in my life right now. My present is free of any negative influences of my past.

Today, I am focused on creating an exciting future. I concern myself with new challenges, rather than the old. When I am free of my past, I get more enjoyment out of my present moments.

Self Reflecting Questions

How does accepting the past help me move forward?

What can I learn from my past challenges?

What items from my past would be best to release from my attention?

What do I gain by focusing on the present and future?

How do I distinguish between letting go and giving up?

Where can I find the courage to stop clinging to things just because they are familiar?

Puzzle #3
POSITIVE FEELINGS

```
S T K G Q L K J T N A I D A R
A R N G R A C I O U S J M S N
T A H E A L T H Y V A X S V I
I N I N S X A N I Q I N K E P
S Q X U K E S C A Z W A I L S
F U I I T X R T I L Q B L T P
I I F N M V R P U G I K L E I
E L T E S P R E E D A B F Y R
D U Z Z A P R E L U I M U K I
D M N U L R I E N A Q O L J T
E I V P V S L R S E X I U W E
G N I V L O V E I S R E N S D
P O I S E D O C S N I E D U T
L U F D N I M Z U S G V S Y J
H S O P T I M I S T I C E J W
```

EVOLVING	JUBILANT	RELAXED
FEARLESS	LUMINOUS	SATISFIED
GENUINE	MAGICAL	SERENE
GRACIOUS	MINDFUL	SKILLFUL
HEALTHY	OPTIMISTIC	SPIRITED
IMPRESSIVE	POISED	STUDIOUS
INSPIRING	PRESENT	SVELTE
JOVIAL	RADIANT	TRANQUIL

Now we know, that your self-concept is basically how you see yourself. But one thing that influences your self-concept, is your self-esteem. Your self-esteem is basically how you feel about yourself or how you personally value, you.

They say that the higher your self-esteem is, the higher your self-concept will be. But the simple fact is, that the world will only see the person that you believe you are. If you walk around with your head down and thinking lowly of yourself, that's exactly how people will receive you. So let's look at some ways that we can boost our self-esteem.

1. Guarantee success by starting small. Success breeds confidence and self-esteem. Create small successes in your life. Drink water instead of soda at lunch. Pay all of your bills on time this month. Any little thing that would make you feel good about yourself is a great place to start.

2. Do something that frightens you. Afraid of dogs? Make a visit to the dog kennel. Afraid of public speaking? Tell a story to several friends simultaneously. Prove to yourself that you can stretch beyond your current comfort zone.

3. Show off your strengths. Are you a great athlete? Sign up for a softball team. Get out and show your stuff. It feels good to do something that you do well. Remind yourself of how skilled and competent you can be. This will boost your confidence and sense of self-esteem. It's enjoyable to show off a little, too.

4. Do something for others. When you help someone else, you feel good about yourself. Deep down, the average person worries about being selfish or inconsiderate. Do something for someone else and you'll convince yourself that you're a good person.

5. Eat a healthier diet. When you eat poorly, you don't feel good. You don't realize how bad you feel. You're just used to it. Your mood and outlook on life will improve when you improve your diet.

6. Avoid comparisons. There's always someone else smarter, better looking, wealthier, or more charismatic. There are a lot of people in the world. Notice the progress you're making in your life and be happy with that.

> We always choose exceptional people to compare ourselves to. So yes, Lupita is better looking and Jeff Bezos is wealthier than you. This will always be true for 99.9999% of the population.

7. Fill your mind with uplifting information. There are plenty of workshops, music, and books with a positive message. With positive information entering your brain on a regular basis, you'll be happier with life and yourself. By the same token, avoid negative information and people.

8. Observe your thoughts. If you pay attention to your thoughts, you'll be both amazed and horrified. It's amazing how your mind jumps around to different topics and the crazy things it thinks. If a real person acted in the same way, you'd call the people in the white coats to come make a pick-up.

- Notice how odd your self-talk can be.

9. Read your affirmations. You should already have a list of affirmations that you believe and keep handy. Whenever you mind is idle, repeat your affirmations to yourself. When you're not busy, your mind will start chattering. Take control of the chatter and keep it positive.

10. Remember your greatness. You've accomplished some impressive things. Make a list of everything you've managed to do in your life up to this point. It's easy to forget how far you've come. Make a list and review it often.

11. Learn something new. Children are so proud of themselves when they learn new things. It might not be as obvious to us as adults, but we experience the same phenomenon. Learn how to bake a cake from scratch or how to hit a golf ball. What interests you? Try to learn a new skill each month.

12. Exercise. You know you're supposed to do it. When you don't do things you know that should be done, you become annoyed with yourself and doubt your self-discipline. Exercise feels good, too. Take care of yourself.

13. Introduce yourself to someone new. This activity carries no risk and has a lot of upside. You feel like you have control over your life, begin to eliminate any shyness, and possibly make a new friend. Everyone fears strangers to some extent. Minimize yours and you'll feel more confident and pleased with yourself.

Puzzle #4

POSITIVE FEELINGS

```
T N E I L L U B E M O S N I W
E V I T I S O P Q K H U W P M
A L G T N E U L F F A G W L F
C H B A N C I R I L C W V E D
D E C O P A C E T I C I A N I
W Z V E N P Y L S Z E A L T L
S C O N S C I O U S M G I I I
C Z K G O P W U U A W P A F G
R E W A R D I N G B O I N U E
B S F G W Z V I B R A N T L N
Q T U I D E L L I F L U F T T
P K L N P U P L I F T E D K Y
N Z E G A S T U T E B R M H E
V D G E L B A R I M D A I R M
D T L D N I K W O R T H Y J S
```

ADMIRABLE	EBULLIENT	REWARDING
AFFLUENT	ENGAGING	UPLIFTED
ASTUTE	FULFILLED	VALIANT
AWAKE	KEEN	VIBRANT
BUOYANT	KIND	WINSOME
CONSCIOUS	NOBLE	WITTY
COPACETIC	PLENTIFUL	WORTHY
DILIGENT	POSITIVE	ZEAL

Low self-esteem can often be traced back to early childhood. For those who had a difficult upbringing or suffered through a traumatic event, low self-esteem is fairly common. However, it's possible to develop self-esteem issues in adulthood as well. When you go through a difficult time, it can affect the way you see yourself.

For example, if you are unemployed, go through a divorce, or file bankruptcy, you may internalize these negative experiences and believe that it's your fault and that you caused these bad things to happen.

Here are some more steps that you can take to overcome low self-esteem:

1. Surround yourself with positive people and remove the negative ones from your life. Spending time with those who are negative will only reinforce your low opinion of yourself. I'm quite sure you heard of the term misery loves company. It's better to surround yourself with individuals who are supportive and encouraging.

* If you're fortunate enough to have positive influences in your life, listen to them when they say you've done a good job.

* Avoid ignoring compliments because you feel unworthy. If you were undeserving of the praise, you wouldn't be getting it.

2. Avoid telling yourself you "should have," "could have," or "would have." If you're constantly telling yourself "I could have done this," or "I should have done that," you're focusing on things that have already happened and that you're unable to change.

* It's better to look to the future and say, "Next time I'll do this," or "I'm going to do that."

3. Set reasonable expectations. Accept that human beings make mistakes. If you're unwilling to accept anything less than perfection from yourself, you'll feel completely discouraged when you inevitably make a mistake.

* Avoid letting mistakes get you down. Remember that every mistake you make is an opportunity to learn and grow.

4. Recognize and celebrate your accomplishments. If your lacking self-esteem, you probably spending a lot of time focusing on the negative. Acknowledge your accomplishments and allow yourself to be happy. It's okay to be proud of yourself.

5. Volunteer for a charitable organization. Working to help others will make you feel good about yourself and help boost your self-esteem.

* It's difficult to have a poor opinion of yourself when you're supporting a good cause.

6. Make a list of all your best qualities. Get a pen and paper and write down your strengths, skills, talents, and positive personality traits.

* When people have low self-esteem, they often focus on all of the things they dislike about themselves. Taking some time to focus on your good qualities can have a very positive effect.

7. Consider seeking professional help. In more extreme cases, low self-esteem can have a negative impact on a person's life and mental health.

* A person with very low self-esteem may have issues in their relationships, trouble in their careers, or a number of other challenges. Sometimes esteem issues can lead to anxiety, social withdrawal, depression, or even suicide.

Puzzle #5

POSITIVE SELF ESTEEM

```
R  E  H  I  N  D  I  V  I  D  U  A  L  P  U
E  S  N  E  T  N  I  D  A  D  E  P  T  F  B
S  L  F  T  S  P  O  N  T  A  N  E  O  U  S
P  I  T  W  E  D  I  R  E  C  T  E  G  N  T
O  Y  E  N  C  R  E  G  D  N  Q  V  B  N  N
N  F  I  L  A  P  P  T  E  C  G  M  R  Y  L
S  M  X  B  B  V  L  R  T  B  J  A  M  N  Q
I  E  O  P  C  A  R  A  I  I  Q  O  G  J  T
V  I  R  D  T  I  D  E  Y  S  M  D  A  E  M
E  U  P  B  E  A  T  N  S  F  I  M  Q  E  D
M  Z  Q  T  P  S  U  S  E  B  U  N  O  B  P
E  V  I  T  I  U  T  N  I  P  O  L  G  C  A
S  G  O  A  E  V  I  T  I  T  E  P  M  O  C
P  A  S  S  I  O  N  A  T  E  R  D  Z  F  D
L  O  Y  A  L  C  H  A  N  G  E  A  B  L  E
```

ADEPT	ENTERPRISING	PASSIONATE
ARTISTIC	FUNNY	PLAYFUL
CHANGEABLE	INDIVIDUAL	RESPONSIVE
COMMITTED	INTENSE	SPONTANEOUS
COMPETITIVE	INTUITIVE	UPBEAT
DEPENDABLE	LOYAL	
DIRECT	MODEST	
ENGAGED	OBSERVANT	

* If low self-esteem is causing chaos in your work and personal life, you may want to consider seeing a therapist for additional help. They can provide you with additional strategies for increasing your self-esteem. A therapist may even be able to help you deal with the underlying issues that caused your low self-esteem in the first place.

There are many factors which can be the root cause or contribute to low self-esteem. The key is to figure out how to overcome your low self-esteem and start feeling good about yourself again, & one of the best ways to do so, is through affirmations!

> Here are a few positive affirmations to get you started, but you can also use these to create your own.

I increase my self-esteem by focusing on my positive qualities.

I can overcome self-doubt and turn it into self-esteem with the power of my mind. I will recall my recent accomplishments and make mental notes of my past achievements. I notice how I handle a variety of situations, and I am proud of my successes.

My self-confidence grows each time I make a healthy and positive choice in my life. I am building a better personal world.

By making a list of my good qualities, I become more aware of how each one is boosting my confidence. I am a strong soul with many positive aspects that make me a special part of the universe.

I have the support of family and friends as I work on boosting my confidence. They are my biggest fans and can help me identify my good qualities.

I am able to live free of comparisons to others and their lives. I am content with my current situation and abilities. I have replaced perfectionism with reality, so I know what to expect from myself.

I let go of anger and negativity because they only stifle my confidence.

Today, I raise my self-esteem by recognizing my talents, strengths, and abilities. I am the only one in the world that has these particular qualities. They make me truly special

My self-esteem comes from acknowledging every achievement.

I acknowledge every one of my accomplishments. I believe everything I achieve is worth recognition. It makes me feel happy and proud when I recognize my successes.

Reminding myself of my accomplishments helps to build my self-esteem. On days when I feel dissatisfied with myself, I take a step back and consider all the positive things I have done in my life.

When I take that approach, I am pleasantly surprised, even by my minor triumphs. Small victories propel me to keep going after higher ones.

I gain self-confidence when I see what I can do. I am my biggest motivator.

I take great pride in my ability to meet deadlines. It proves that I am reliable. I know that I am valuable to others when I am reliable. My employer has great confidence in me because of my track record.

When I support my loved ones, I feel accomplished. I know that my support helps them to keep moving forward in a positive direction.

I find something to be proud of even when I achieve less than I expect. I take the time to learn from those situations. Learning builds my confidence because then I know that I can do better the next time.

Today, my self-esteem pushes me to achieve great things. I believe in myself because I acknowledge every success along the way. Seeing what I can do gives me the drive to go reach higher goals in life.

Puzzle #6
POSITIVE SELF ESTEEM

```
L Q D H Z X D G H C F N C G F
J Z H V Y N Z M G O N A I N A
E L B A I C O S A A N A D Q C
K K V H S Z L C I T C E L C E
P E R S I S T E N T U H S L A
X I L D I R E C T E J R J T W
E M N Y G D U R Y N L C E T T
Y L D N E I R F T T V M U E S
G T F A O C O E V I T A E R C
G J E M A V O N Z V V L R C M
E U Q I N U A U V E W E U Y C
B P T C E V I T A N I G A M I
L R Z P S H E V I T C E J B O
N R E L I A B L E V O S L P K
H J J M O T I V A T E D H F L
```

ASSERTIVE	IMAGINATIVE	UNIQUE
ATTENTIVE	INNOVATIVE	
CREATIVE	MATURE	
DIRECT	MOTIVATED	
DYNAMIC	OBJECTIVE	
ECLECTIC	PERSISTENT	
FRIENDLY	RELIABLE	
HONEST	SOCIABLE	

Everyone can benefit from a little more self-esteem. When you think more highly of yourself, you're in a better position to change your self-concept and your life. Think of more ways to boost your self-esteem and continue to apply these concepts daily.

When you love yourself you never feel the need to justify to the world or those around you, when or why you treat yourself the way you do. You feel a sense of freedom and empowerment when you do things to add value to your life.

For your Homework: Make one small, positive change to your daily routine starting tomorrow. Keep it small and simple, but make sure that it is something positive that adds to your life and the person you are becoming. By doing so your self-esteem will begin to grow day by day.

Self-Reflection Questionnaire

1. What are the limiting beliefs I hold that were created through past experiences?

2. Are these limiting beliefs valid? Where did they come from? Is it possible I interpreted the situation incorrectly?

3. How is my current life limiting my beliefs about myself, my capabilities, and my ability to control my future and my environment?

4. How can I learn to better appreciate and recognize my own abilities?

5. Am I always honest with myself regarding achievements?

6. How do I handle situations where someone tries to discredit my achievement?

7. How important is the support of family and friends to my self-esteem?

8. Do others see some positive qualities in me that I haven't recognized? What are they?

9. What can I do to avoid comparing my life with the accomplishments of others?

Self-Reflection Questionnaire

10. What changes do I need to make to my finances, health, and social life to support a more effective self-concept?

11. Who do I want to become? Who do I admire?

12. What can I do today to begin living more like the person I want to be?

13. On a scale of 1-10 how would I rate my self-esteem?

14. What are the biggest barriers to feeling better about myself?

15. What can I do to overcome those barriers?

Puzzle #7
POSITIVE SELF ESTEEM

```
X E N D B M T E N A C I O U S
T C V O A R E A L I S T I C U
L C F I P N E T G Q V W R C C
P O X D T T A F H P T S X J C
V N V J E A I L L O G S V F E
C F G I A T R M Y E D O W V S
V I B N B R T O I T C I C L S
Z D T T O R T I B S I T C T F
Q E U E I R A I M A T C I A U
U N D N H R T N C M L I A V L
W T V S M T G S T U O L C L E
O B S E R V A N T G L C O O R
T L U F T C E P S E R A Z C X
T A L E N T E D M P H Z T L E
C I N T E L L I G E N T N E G
```

ANALYTICAL   METHODICAL   TALENTED
ARTICULATE   OBSERVANT   TENACIOUS
COLLABORATIVE OPTIMISTIC   VIBRANT
COMMITTED   REALISTIC
CONFIDENT   REFLECTIVE
EMPATHETIC   RESPECTFUL
INTELLIGENT   STRONG
INTENSE   SUCCESSFUL

Redefining Your Self Through Conscious Awareness

Have you ever felt like you're just going through the motions? You get up, go to work, come home, maybe have dinner, watch television, and go to bed. The next day, you start the routine all over again.

But what if I told you, that you can become more connected with your own experiences? And that by doing so, you would enjoy life more, feel happier and more content, and have more control over your life. Well guess what, by living consciously, you can live that type of life!

All you have to do is make a decision to do so!

So what does it actually mean to live Consciously?

Living consciously simply means, being aware and responsible for your life. Responsible for your actions, responsible for your thoughts, responsible for the words that come out of your mouth, responsible for what you put in your mouth, and the things you allow to enter your life.

Living consciously means that you live life fully aware of your actions and reactions to everyone and thing around you. You recognize that every thing you do has a consequence, whether it is positive or negative. You acknowledge that whatever you are reaping in life is in direct relation to the seeds that you have previously sown, and that things just don't happen. That you create your destiny, you may not have dealt the hand you have, but playing & winning, is solely up to you.

So how do we begin to life on a conscious level daily?

So now that you know what it means to live life consciously, how do we do it successfully. Well, in order to live a fulfilling life, you have to be totally in control of your psyche. Remember you are in the drivers seat, now that doesn't mean that you are in total control. Even a farmer has to have faith in a higher power, he can not control the sun and the rain, and doesn't necessarily know or understand exactly, how a seed turns into fruit, but he obeys the laws of nature and does his part.

In the same way we have to acknowledge that there are laws, that we can not change, but that are designed to benefit us in life, and if we utilize them to our advantage, we too can partake in an abundance of harvests, as long as we sow faithfully.

Now for the most part, you may still have to get up in the morning, go to work, return home, eat supper and so on, but the difference now would be, that you do it with a purpose.

You can simply begin by asking yourself, what do you really want in life, is your goal to just merely survive. What are you actually working for or towards. If your goal is to just keep a roof over your head and food in your belly. I would say you are missing the point of life. We were not designed to serve each other. Or to be subject to only making someone else's life or business better. We all have something that the world needs.

We all have gifts and a major purpose, and as long as you remain unconscious to your purpose, you will never be able to live a fulfilling life.

Thinking consciously enables you to discover, that you have the control in your life to do whatever it is that brings you joy, pleasure, and contentment.

Living consciously empowers you to cease wasting time doing activities you're not really interested in. When you make a personal vow to live consciously, you're opening the door to a new, more joyous existence.

You can start by asking yourself theses simple questions:

* What are you truly seeking in life?
* With whom do you choose to spend most of your time with?
* How can you spend leisure time in ways that re-charge you and excite joy?
* How can you become more psychologically engaged in your work to increase your performance?
* Are you taking care of your physical self the way you want and obtaining the results you desire?

Your answers to these questions will lead you down the path of conscious living.

Go ahead and take the first step in your journey toward reclaiming your life today. Say to yourself: "I will live consciously every moment today." Repeat it tomorrow and the day after and embrace the joys of creating the life you desire.

From now on as you do your routine tasks throughout the day, concentrate on what you're doing. Always ask yourself, are you doing your best? Or is it a more effective or efficient method to get the task or project done?

Puzzle #8
REASONS WHY I LOVE ME

```
L U F I T U A E B F D I M P W
S T D E R I P S N I H N Q X G
M Y P P A H P W W U E D I O R
A U G Z K R G D O D A E C K A
R D T G F M L P U K L P T W T
T A E P N V A E W B T E H O E
A N Y T H I N G S V H N A N F
L E E V A O H R I S Y D N D U
J O V D Y C N T E C D E K E L
V J V I I E U E Y M D N F R V
G C D E T F N D S R A T U F V
Z A Y Y D A N R E T E E L U J
C O U R A G E O U S G V R L X
F I B P Z Q U R C O Q B E D L
E L B I S S O P C Y J W J I E
```

ANYTHING	FEARLESS	KIND
BEAUTIFUL	GRATEFUL	LOVED
CONFIDENT	HAPPY	MAGIC
COURAGEOUS	HEALTHY	POSSIBLE
CREATIVE	HONEST	SMART
DREAMER	INDEPENDENT	THANKFUL
EDUCATED	INSPIRED	WONDERFUL
EVERYTHING	JOURNEY	

Now, another way to enhance your self-concept is to make some positive changes. It's much easier to think positively about yourself when you have an enjoyable and successful life

Generally speaking, I guess there's nothing inherently wrong with living in a shoe box, eating instant soup every night, and being 50lbs over weight.. However, happy thoughts are easier to come by when you're pleased with yourself and your life!

Consider the main parts of your life and ask yourself are you happy. But let's look at a few areas in life that you may be neglecting or need to improve.

Health and Well-Being

Are you as healthy and fit as you'd like to be? Although you may not desire to have a 6-pack to show off at the beach, but being healthy has its advantages. Good health should be a high priority for anyone that values them self. An attractive body also boosts self-esteem and demonstrates to you that you can control yourself.

Prove to yourself that you're worth the time and energy to maintain good health:

1. See your physician for a checkup. Everyone should see the doctor at least once per year. There are plenty of health conditions that don't always show obvious symptoms, yet are very serious. Diabetes, hypertension, and high cholesterol are just a few examples.

    - Taking care of yourself demonstrates your belief that you're valuable and relevant. An "I don't care" attitude demonstrates the total opposite.

2. Exercise regularly. Everyone needs to exercise, bottom line. There is No reason not to exercise. Exercising promotes health and extends our lives.

3. Find and maintain a healthy weight. No one enjoys being overweight, and it can be a serious challenge to one's self-esteem. However, it's also challenging to change your bodyweight for the better in the long-term.

- Make small nutritional changes that you can maintain. Eliminating a can of soda each day and substituting water is one such change.
- When you maintain a healthy weight, your life is just easier. You process and eliminate foods better and it's less stress overall on your body. Did you know for every pound of extra weight you carry it transfers to five extra pounds on your knees, which in turn puts more weight on your ankles and increases your chance of injury or joint damage.

Your overall goal in life should be, to be as healthy as possible. Eat a healthy diet, get some exercise, and see your doctor regularly. Take good care of yourself. You're worth it.

"Never rely on your spouse, family, career, Dr. or anyone else for your happiness, health or self-worth. Only you can be responsible for that. If you don't love and respect yourself – no one else will be able to make that happen for you. Accept the person that you are – completely; and if you are Not happy with the good and the bad – then make the necessary changes as YOU see fit – and not because you think someone else thinks or wants you to be different."

Social Life

No one is an island. We are all social creatures, so unless your dream is to become a hermit, it's necessary to involve others in your life. Your self-concept is affected by the quality of your social life. If you wish there were more people interested in spending time with you, become the person that you would like to spend time with.

You can start enjoying a more fulfilling social life at any moment by starting to follow just a few simple steps:

1. Decide on the type of social life you would like to create. Not everyone wants to be the life of the party and spend time with a different bunch of people every night. Maybe you'd rather have a couple of close friends that you meet for coffee twice a week and a regular social activity on the weekend. It's up to you. Or maybe a little of both, think about it.

2. Figure out what has been the limiting factor to you living this life already. When you know the cause, you can make a plan. A few possibilities include:

    ○ I work at home and don't have regular contact with others.
    ○ I'm shy.
    ○ I don't know what, to actually say to people

3. Create and implement a solution. There are books on how to be more charismatic. You can find videos on how to get over social anxiety or how to deal with shyness. Maybe you need to reach out to the people you already know. Perhaps you can join a club or start a new hobby that involves other people.

* You can begin to build your social life one person at a time. Most people only need a couple of good friends to feel satisfaction and self-esteem in this part of their lives.

You can also look for new friends in places where you frequent, like work, your neighborhood, the coffee shop, or grocery store, or try getting in touch with old friends, or joining meet-ups.

Creating an enjoyable social life is much easier than you think. Always remember that most people are only lonely in the areas, that they choose to be. We are all social beings, it's not that hard to find others that would like to get out of the house and share a meaningful activity or conversation.

Puzzle #9

SELF ESTEEM

```
X S S E N M L A C I T C A R P
E R U S A E L P O W E R F U L
T U D I N V E N T I V E W P D
H U M I L I T Y D Z Z Z W R I
O A C E X C I T I N G A M O Z
U E P O D T H R G U X E Z D F
G A C P M E E K N E S S E U B
H E I N I P M G I J U Z R C R
T E H C E N O C T G P Z E T H
F V S O S D E S Y L R R W I Y
U T P F N L I S U C I W Y V K
L L P M F O N F S R D V B E Q
G Z A S S U R A N C E J B E Y
V A L U E Y V M M O D E S T Y
S M O R A L E V I T C A O R P
```

ASSURANCE	HUMILITY	PRIDE
CALMNESS	INVENTIVE	PROACTIVE
COMPOSURE	MEEKNESS	PRODUCTIVE
CONFIDENCE	MODESTY	THOUGHTFUL
DIGNITY	MORALE	VALUE
EXCITING	PLEASURE	
HAPPINESS	POWERFUL	
HONOR	PRACTICAL	

Finances

It's hard to be pleased with yourself if you're filling your gas tank $5 at a time. Having the ability to pay for life's basic necessities is important to your self-concept. It's easy to think negatively about yourself when you can't manage your own expenses.

Managing your finances:

1. Create a budget and stick to it. Whether you earn $30,000 or $3 million, we all need a budget. There are numerous websites and books dedicated to personal finance and budgeting. Learn the fundamentals of budgeting, it's part of being an adult.

2. Develop an attitude to save. A proper budget will provide for an excess of funds at the end of each month. Save the excess and then look for ways to invest it appropriately.

3. Then begin to look for ways to Earn more. If you are not meeting your expenses with your current income, the only solution is to either cut expenses or earn more.

4. There are several ways to increase your income:

    - Find a second job.
    - Get a raise at your current job.
    - Find a better paying job.
    - Create a primary or secondary job for yourself. There are numerous opportunities online in today's world.

Think about the type of future you want & the financial life that appeals to you and begin immediately to take the steps to make it happen. Money isn't everything, but it is highly relevant. You'll feel more accomplished and less discouragement if your financial life is healthy.

Now once you've created your budget and have started managing your finances, start creating new goals!

Do you currently have any goals? Being excited about the future and making consistent progress in life will dramatically enhance your concept of yourself.

Numerous studies have shown that people with goals outperform the rest of the population in every area of life. Having a few goals creates a sense of purpose, direction, and self-control.

Puzzle #10

SELF ESTEEM

```
G L Y T C A P A B L E R F Z P
B R I L L I A N T E N N Q E B
A B R S T E T N E T E P M O C
E T F W S C L S R N H S Z W R
N V H Z W E U B I E H G V I V
J D I L K B N L A U S N I O D
E M O S E W A L T T R P I R B
W I K J I T S G L U P T E Z B
O R X I P C I I N E R A L C S
R T N Q C E E C S I W E D A T
T Z G U B H L D D E R O D A J
H O A U T H E N T I C U P W R
Y E L B A M I T S E D S L S X
W C O M M E N D A B L E A L K
S U O E T R U O C R P Y V Z A
```

ADAPTABLE	BRIGHT	ESTIMABLE
ADORED	BRILLIANT	RESPECT
ALLURING	CAPABLE	WELLNESS
ALTRUISTIC	COMMENDABLE	WORTHY
ASCESIS	COMPETENT	
ATHLETIC	COURTEOUS	
AUTHENTIC	CULTURED	
AWESOME	DECISIVE	

Developing Goals

Creating simple and effective goals:

1. Create S.M.A.R.T. goals with a timeline no longer than 12 weeks. It's hard to maintain focus and enthusiasm longer than this. If your goal is too big to reach in 12 weeks, set short-term goals that will take you in the right direction.

2. Continually examine your progress. This keeps your goals fresh in your mind and provides the feedback you need to maximize your effectiveness.

3. Get excited by progress. If you want to enhance your self-concept, feel good about yourself at every opportunity. Most people have been stuck in the same place for years, so any progress in life is worthy of celebration.

On the next page we break down the acronym S.M.A.R.T. in S.M.A.R.T. goal making and on the following page there is a S.M.A.R.T Goal Checklist with a few extra ones in the back of the book.

Sometimes setting goals can be a stressful and complicated process, but it doesn't have to be. Having a few short term and long term goals and making regular progress can be great for your self-concept. It proves to you that you can make changes in your life whenever you want and ultimately control your future.

SMART Goals

"SMART" is a common goal-setting strategy that you can use when starting a new goal. It helps ensure that your goal is capable of being achieved. Below is a flowchart that will help you determine how realistic it is for you to reach your desired goals.

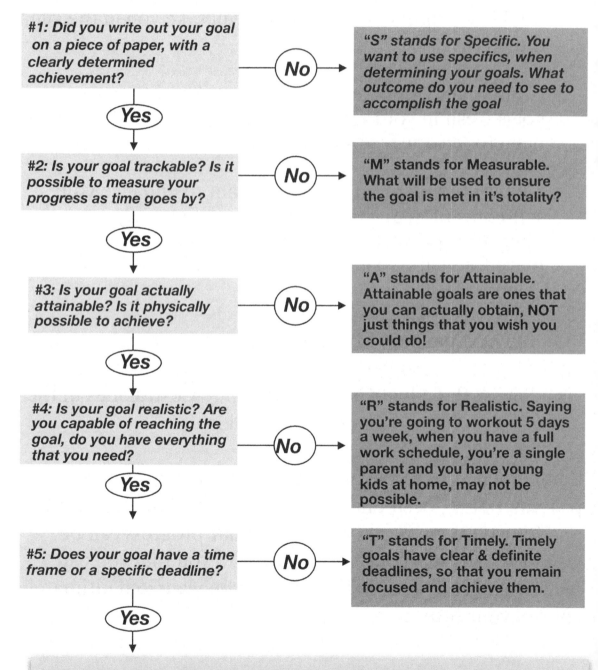

S.M.A.R.T Goal Checklist

S _____

_____

M _____

_____

A _____

_____

R _____

_____

T _____

Goal

_____

_____

_____

_____

Puzzle #11
SELF ESTEEM

```
M  E  T  I  C  U  L  O  U  S  Y  Z  G  P  C
Z  G  L  R  O  T  A  I  T  I  N  I  Y  O  O
I  N  D  U  S  T  R  I  O  U  S  R  J  S  B
K  N  P  E  F  L  E  M  E  N  J  Q  G  I  O
B  T  R  S  P  R  A  U  L  V  U  X  M  T  R
I  E  E  W  E  I  E  C  X  A  I  A  J  I  I
X  R  C  H  K  D  J  E  H  R  C  T  M  V  G
P  F  I  B  M  T  X  T  H  I  E  I  C  E  I
A  B  S  Z  B  A  L  A  N  C  E  D  G  A  N
T  N  E  D  N  E  P  E  D  N  I  V  A  O  A
I  D  I  P  L  O  M  A  T  I  C  R  E  E  L
E  X  X  J  Q  R  O  T  A  I  D  E  M  R  L
N  E  V  I  T  A  R  E  P  O  O  C  R  R  K
T  L  C  E  M  O  T  I  O  N  A  L  O  W  C
N  O  U  T  G  O  I  N  G  T  M  K  F  D  Z
```

ACHIEVER	INDUSTRIOUS	PATIENT
ACTIVE	INITIATOR	POSITIVE
BALANCED	LEADER	PRECISE
CHEERFUL	LOGICAL	
COOPERATIVE	MEDIATOR	
DIPLOMATIC	METICULOUS	
EMOTIONAL	ORIGINAL	
INDEPENDENT	OUTGOING	

Giving of Yourself on a Regular Basis

It's never always all about you. Your self-concept isn't solely about you either. It's also about your perception of your value to the world. Providing value to the world selflessly is the greatest way to prove a change in your self-concept and to boost your self-esteem.

1. Volunteer. Organizations are always looking for more volunteers. Find an organization that appeals to you, or a cause that you can contribute to and get involved.

2. Find a job or second job that gives you the opportunity to help others. You could tutor children or teach adults to read. Maybe you work with senior citizens one night a week in the evenings. There are many jobs available that provide a meaningful service to others.

3. Perform random acts of kindness. Life presents endless opportunities to help others. You can't help but love yourself when you're doing something wonderful for another person.

Helping others when possible will benefit you in many unpredictable ways. Look for opportunities throughout your day to help others. Think about small changes that you could make to be more helpful or kind to others?

You will begin to have a higher opinion of yourself when you're pleased in these simple areas of your life. The more satisfied you are with yourself, the easier it is to be authentic.

For your homework: Create a 12-week S.M.A.R.T. Goal to make one change in one of the areas mentioned in this lesson. Make the goal small enough that you'll find it pretty easy to see success with it.

Write down your goal and remind yourself of your new goal several times each day. But avoid just thinking about it – take actions each day to make it happen.

Here are a few affirmations to get you started:

Each day I strive to become the person I want to be.

I always strive to improve myself. I look forward to learning and accumulating more skills so that I am more productive in all aspects of my life.

Using patience, I am able to be compassionate with others. I show them the kindness they deserve. In all relationships, whether they are personal or professional, I strive to be a person that others can look up to.

I maintain a positive attitude so I can work with situations as they occur and develop effective solutions. I look forward to the future so I can portray even more strength as I go through my life.

When I help others, I learn more about myself. I am always ready to assist others with what they need. When I offer my guidance, I feel proud of myself.

I work to counter my imperfections. Making myself into the person I want to be sometimes seems like a challenge, but I know that I am up to the task.

Today, I am paying extra attention to becoming the person that I want to be. In my professional and personal life, I want to be able to be proud of my actions.

Self-Reflection Questions:

1. What are my goals for self-improvement?
2. What can I do to strengthen my personal relationships?
3. How can I ensure that I am putting in one hundred percent with any endeavor that I set my mind on?

Puzzle #12
SELF LOVE

```
H E A L T H Y K M C D T C N R
S B T T N E U Q O L E M E Q A
L U E I Z S R L V J S I M Y D
L U O N S A C O N O E N P L I
D O F L C I D I L V R D O T A
G E V E U H U G M I V F W I N
R E L I P B A Q B A I U E E T
A F V A N O A N X L N L R G P
C V J O T G H F T E G Y E L P
I U G E L E C T R I C A D O J
O T D S L V D F O W N I Q R Q
U H R D E R I P S N I G D I W
S J U B I L A N T D E S I O P
F T N E S E R P G B K L X U R
H J Z E L I B E R A T E D S Z
```

DESERVING   EXQUISITE   JUBILANT
DYNAMIC   FABULOUS   LIBERATED
ELATED   GLORIOUS   LOVING
ELECTRIC   GRACIOUS   MINDFUL
ELOQUENT   HEALTHY   POISED
EMPOWERED   HOPEFUL   PRESENT
ENCHANTING   INSPIRED   RADIANT
EVOLVING   JOVIAL

Who do you desire to become?

When we begin to create concrete examples of who we want to be, and the qualities in life that we desire to exhibit to the world, it can help foster and inspire us from within. Most people never aspire to be more, than what they see around them. Especially if their parents did not instill proper moral and ethical values in them when they were younger. If all your parents ever told you was to get an education and get a good job, your aspirations may not go beyond a pretty cubicle in the corner of an office at a job that you despise.

But when you begin to live life according to your personal beliefs and desires, your self-concept will begin to flourish.

Make a conscious decision on who you want to be:

1. Who do you admire and why? Do you wish you were more like Angela Merkel? Why? Are you a fan of Marie Curie? Rosa Parks? Why?

2. What personal qualities have you always admired in others?

    - Charisma?
    - Confidence?
    - Mental toughness?
    - Kindness?
    - Cool under pressure?
    - Happiness

3. What can you do today to start becoming the person you've always wanted to be? There's no one that can stop you. Anyone that tries to get in your way can be ignored. Get on a mission to become the person that you desire.

This is your ultimate goal. When you become the person you wish to be and begin living the life you desire, your opinion of yourself will be at the highest possible level. Everything else is just a stepping stone to reach this point.

Even as you begin to work on enhancing your self-concept, it's important to take the time to accept yourself, at every point, no matter where you may be on your journey.

Now time for your Homework:

Go to your journal, and write down one quality that you admire in someone else. What will it take for you to begin to start demonstrating this quality yourself? Make a conscious decision to yourself, to spend the required time to practice doing it each day.

Now before we end this chapter of your life and start on the new one, there is one important thing that we have to resolve in regards to our past.

Puzzle #13

UNIQUE SELF WORTH

```
Z L O S L A C I T I L O P E P
C P R E U X D D N P N P V S E
V G G E V I T A N I G A M I R
P X A W Q L U F P L E H P N S
E P N P E R C E P T I V E C O
R D I J E L B A I M A W S E N
S K Z N W P O F S L M B O R A
U R E N D P D E T H B R L E B
A F D E G S Q Q L Z I T I E L
S Y O Y F E S I W B T X D L E
I G T C S E N S I T I V E E L
V M N T U U Q U C M O X B G O
E V V V I S U O I R U C E R I
D K J B J W E S E N S I B L E
E S K I L L E D N B E H O H F
```

ADAPTABLE
AMBITIOUS
AMIABLE
CURIOUS
FLEXIBLE
FOCUSED
GENUINE
HELPFUL

IMAGINATIVE
ORGANIZED
PERCEPTIVE
PERSONABLE
PERSUASIVE
PERSUASIVE
POLITICAL
SENSIBLE

SENSITIVE
SINCERE
SKILLED
SOLID
WISE
WITTY

Breaking Away from Self-Limiting Thought Patterns

Now one of the biggest hinderances in your efforts to live, learn, and grow is negative thought patterns or habits. By now you have realized how your personal beliefs about yourself and your life effect your future or we can say past as of today. In fact, those beliefs became the very foundation upon which you built the life you are currently living.

But now you are equipped with tools to change your life, but remember it is a process, and that old foundation is not going to just disappear. So let's look at some ways that it may choose to pop up and sabotage your plans in the future.

So how do you recognize self-sabotaging thoughts?

Some common self-limiting thoughts are:

* "I'll never be able to save any money for retirement."
* "I guess I won't ever fall in love again."
* "Why can't I find any trustworthy friends?"
* "I'll be fat forever."
* "I'm sure Tammy will get that promotion over me."
* "I wish I could take a vacation to Aruba, but I know I could never afford it."
* "How will I ever live the life I want earning what I earn now?"

If you could identify with any of those limiting thoughts while reading the above examples, immediately begin to take the necessary steps to break your cognitive ties to those thinking patterns.

Here are a few strategies to get you started thinking in a new direction:

1. Refrain from labeling yourself. If you see yourself as "broke" financially, then you might unconsciously strive to match that label. Or if you think of yourself as "big boned" you may be unable to imagine yourself as beautiful and thin.

2. Take baby steps. When you begin continually moving towards your goals, you'll gain the momentum to keep on going. Rather than thinking you're unable to achieve success, make a plan of achievable steps to ensure you do.

* For example, perhaps you'd like a Caribbean vacation. Instead of believing you'll never get there, establish a small weekly savings goal of a specific amount, and keep putting the money aside until you have enough.

3. Learn to be your own best friend. Love yourself enough to be your own best friend. Do this by giving yourself the benefit of the doubt. Think positive thoughts such as, "I can do this." When you practice this, you'll reject self-limiting thoughts.

4. Believe in yourself. Instead of insisting you'll "never" do something, say that you can, and then do it. If you turn those negatives into positives, it boosts your self-esteem. Trust that you can accomplish, succeed, and prevail anything you set out to do.

5. Constantly Assess the truth. Ask yourself, "Is what I'm thinking really true?" For example, is it an absolute reality that you'll never be able to save any money at all for retirement? It doesn't have to be true, unless you believe it.

* Immediately change your mindset by beginning your retirement fund today. At the end of every day, put all of your change and single dollars into a jar. See how simple it is to start saving?

* Question your self-limiting thoughts. When you realize they're unrealistic, untrue, and within your power to change, you'll be able to break away.

6. Recognize how powerful your negative thoughts are. You create who you are by what you think about yourself. Why not turn that power into positive energy that drives you towards the things that you want in life?

7. Learn from prior errors. Instead of using your past against you, think about the knowledge you've gained from each experience. Maybe an important relationship dissolved a few years ago. The loss of that relationship doesn't mean you'll never find another partner again.

* Rather than tearing yourself down with self-limiting thoughts, reflect on the shortcomings of your previous relationship. What part did you play? If you proactively learn from your past mistakes, you'll make healthier choices in the future.

When you apply the above strategies to your life, you'll see the possibilities that are all around you. You can do anything you set your mind to. Extinguish those self-limiting beliefs right now so you can start embracing the good life that's yours for the taking.

Puzzle #14

VALUES

```
G T V J G N I T S E R E T N I
J N N I E G D E L W O N K F E
S C I A L F N E V O L F L E S
E T J W G U K I N D N E S S M
L H B I O E F D T W O H Z N P
F R A S W L L P Z I E O A T Y
A I M H A N G E L I C A C Y Z
W L N F U G B V L E A X L N K
A L S U J E R M U Q H D E T S
R E X L A D V E N T U R E M H
E D W U A U T H E N T I C P Z
C I F I R R E T A A A S I B T
N Y L T P M O R P K B J P R V
S S E C C U S M E V O L Y J I
D E T A V I T O M E A G E R J
```

ADEPT	GLOWING	PROMPTLY
ADVENTURE	HELPFUL	SELF AWARE
AGREEABLE	INTERESTING	SELF LOVE
ANGELIC	KINDNESS	SUCCESS
AUTHENTIC	KNOWLEDGE	TERRIFIC
EAGER	LOVE	THRILLED
ELEGANT	MORALS	WEALTH
EXCITING	MOTIVATED	WISHFUL

Summary & Reflection

So now that you have realized that your self-concept has been shaped by your past. Or rather, your perception of it, and you have reviewed all of the uncomfortable experiences from your past and have hopefully found a few positive resolutions. I just want to remind you one more time, that the past is only a limitation if you allow it to be.

With your renewed self-esteem you have the fuel to continue making alterations to your self-concept. This is an ongoing process. You already have plenty of reasons to be happy with yourself. Ensure you remind yourself of how wonderful you already are daily, continue utilizing and rewriting your affirmations.

Be proactive about enhancing your life according to your own wishes. By continuously creating and living the life you desire, your self-concept will continue to grow and change. When you begin to have evidence that you're living your idea of a happy life, take the time to embrace where you are, but never get complacent, there always areas where you can continue to grow and become better.

You are authentic and you should be proud to present yourself to the world just the way you are!

Puzzle #15

WHY I LOVE ME

```
U G T N E T S I S R E P N Q Z
O E L B A R O N O H N A H W R
J N L P A T I E N C E J A P E
G E O B Y T I R G E T N I X S
V R Q A O T C M D W W F W J I
T O A I C N I R A E O A C L
R U G T N C N S Z X R I B R I
U S O N I N O A O H K T I E E
S N W P I T O U F I E H B P N
T Q O M T R U V N W R F L U C
I M V I A I U D A T G U I T E
N I S K S H M T E T A L C A K
G U V J E S F I R V I B A B V
Y T I R U T A M S U I V L L O
G Y F Q K P E P F M N L E E Q
```

ACCOUNTABLE   INTEGRITY   PERSISTENT
BIBLICAL   MATURITY   REPUTABLE
CURIOSITY   NETWORKER   RESILIENCE
FAITHFUL   NOBLE   TRUSTING
GENEROUS   NURTURING
GRATITUDE   OPTIMISM
HONORABLE   PASSION
INNOVATIVE   PATIENCE

Puzzle #16

WHY I LOVE ME

```
O  P  P  O  R  T  U  N  I  T  Y  G  R  N  J
Z  P  R  E  S  T  I  G  E  R  U  T  U  F  V
T  B  R  A  V  E  Y  L  I  M  A  F  N  A  H
V  D  E  M  D  B  K  G  R  P  W  G  Y  B  U
C  I  P  A  R  I  S  T  O  C  R  A  T  I  C
B  O  S  G  U  R  L  Y  B  L  F  L  F  R  F
F  H  L  R  I  T  N  I  A  T  O  L  Z  T  F
R  I  D  L  E  H  Y  O  G  D  B  I  B  H  R
I  S  K  R  E  D  G  T  I  E  I  L  B  R  E
E  T  V  F  K  A  L  X  R  T  N  L  T  I  E
N  O  B  A  X  Y  G  E  X  E  A  C  O  G  D
D  R  S  T  E  S  N  U  S  Z  B  C  E  H  O
S  Y  B  Z  C  E  F  V  E  C  F  I  U  T  M
E  Y  T  I  L  I  B  I  S  S  O  P  L  D  O
U  N  P  V  E  R  U  T  L  U  C  J  L  W  E
```

ARISTOCRATIC	DILIGENCE	HOLIDAYS
BEAUTY	EDUCATION	LIBERTY
BIOLOGY	ELDERS	OPPORTUNITY
BIRTHDAYS	FAMILY	POSSIBILITY
BIRTHRIGHT	FREEDOM	PRESTIGE
BRAVE	FRIENDS	SUNSETS
COLLEAGUES	FUTURE	
CULTURE	HISTORY	

S.M.A.R.T Goal Checklist

S

M

A

R

T

Goal

S.M.A.R.T Goal Checklist

S

M

A

R

T

Goal

S.M.A.R.T Goal Checklist

S

M

A

R

T

Goal

S.M.A.R.T Goal Checklist

(S) _____

(M) _____

(A) _____

(R) _____

(T) _____

Goal

S.M.A.R.T Goal Checklist

S

M

A

R

T

Goal

My Self-Concept Journal

Positive Affirmation

Positive Affirmation

Positive Affirmation

_____
_____
_____
_____

Positive Affirmation

Positive Affirmation

_____
_____
_____
_____
_____

_____
_____
_____
_____
_____

Positive Affirmation

Positive Affirmation

Positive Affirmation

Positive Affirmation

Positive Affirmation

Positive Affirmation

Positive Affirmation

Positive Affirmation

Positive Affirmation

Positive Affirmation

Positive Affirmation

Positive Affirmation

Positive Affirmation

Positive Affirmation

Positive Affirmation

Positive Affirmation

Positive Affirmation

Positive Affirmation

Positive Affirmation

(Positive Affirmation)

(Positive Affirmation)

(Positive Affirmation)

○ Positive Affirmation

○ Positive Affirmation

○ Positive Affirmation

Self-Concept Quiz Answers

Quiz 1: Answer Key

1. a
2. d
3. b
4. a
5. d

Quiz 2: Answer Key

1. a
2. b
3. a
4. d
5. b

I AM PUZZLE
Puzzle # 1

```
   E V I T A E R C L A Y O L
     G D N   O     T B       P
E     E N E A   P   T   L P A
N L     V I C I   E E       E S
T   B T D I V I L   N     A S
H A T I N E T R S L T   H C I
U L T N X E N A E I I   U E O
S T U T E E D I I S V R M F N
I R   F R C L I M C E E B U A
A U     E A O F F R E D L L T
S S E     P C N   N E R E   E
T T   S     O T N   O T P
I I     I     H I I   C E P
C N       W C L E V E R   D A
  G     C O U R A G E O U S
```

I COULD BE
Puzzle # 2

```
            J O U R N A L I S T
P H Y S I C I A N U         O
R J U D G E   R       R       R
N E     R   T   E     S     T
U A T     O   E   E       E H
T   I H T T S Y L A N A   O L
R O T C G C N S   H   I   D A
I N L U I I E A E   T   G O W
T   O I A R F T T F   A   N Y
I M   E P N T E I N O     T E
O A   G   O C R H U R     I R
N Y     R   R E I C O P S
I O       U   T L F R C T
S R       S   S E   A C
T     T S I C A M R A H P     A
```

POSITIVE FEELINGS
Puzzle # 3

```
S T             J T N A I D A R
A R N G R A C I O U S       S
T A H E A L T H Y V     S V
I N   N S   A N     I   K E
S Q   U   E S C A       A I L S
F U I I     R T I L     L T P
I I F N M   R P U G I   L E I
E L   E S P   E E D A B F   R
D U     A P R E L U I M U   I
  M       R I E N A Q O L J T
    I       L R S E X I U   E
G N I V L O V E I S R E N S D
P O I S E D       S N I E D U
L U F D N I M     S G V S
    S O P T I M I S T I C E
```

POSITIVE FEELINGS
Puzzle # 4

```
T N E I L L U B E M O S N I W
E V I T I S O P     K     P
  L   T N E U L F F A     L
    B   N         W V E D
    C O P A C E T I C   A N I
      E N   Y     Z E A L T L
C O N S C I O U S       I I I
Z   G         U   W   A F G
R E W A R D I N G B     I N U E
S   G       V I B R A N T L N
T     I D E L L I F L U F T T
K   N   U P L I F T E D     Y
    E G A S T U T E
      E L B A R I M D A
      D N I K W O R T H Y
```

POSITIVE SELF ESTEEM
Puzzle # 5

R	E		I	N	D	I	V	I	D	U	A	L	
E	S	N	E	T	N	I		A	D	E	P	T	F
S			T	S	P	O	N	T	A	N	E	O	U	S
P		T		E	D	I	R	E	C	T		N	
O		E	N		R	E		N				N	
N			L	A	P	P	T			G		Y	
S	M			B	V	L	R	T		A			
I		O		C	A	R	A	I	I		G		
V			D		I	D	E	Y	S	M		E	
E	U	P	B	E	A	T	N	S	F	I	M		D
				S		S	E	B	U	N	O		
E	V	I	T	I	U	T	N	I	P	O	L	G	C
				E	V	I	T	I	T	E	P	M	O	C
P	A	S	S	I	O	N	A	T	E	R	D		
L	O	Y	A	L	C	H	A	N	G	E	A	B	L	E

POSITIVE SELF ESTEEM
Puzzle # 6

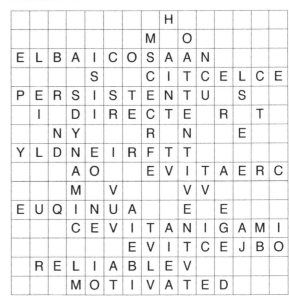

POSITIVE SELF ESTEEM
Puzzle # 7

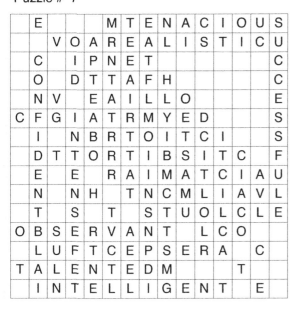

REASONS WHY I LOVE ME
Puzzle # 8

L	U	F	I	T	U	A	E	B		D	I			
S		D	E	R	I	P	S	N	I	H	N			G
M	Y	P	P	A	H				E	D	I			R
A				R				A	E		K	A
R	D		G		M	L			L	P	T	W	T
T		E		N		A	E		T	E	H	O	E
A	N	Y	T	H	I	N	G	S		H	N	A	N	F
L	E	E			A	O	H	R	I	S	Y	D	N	D	U
O	V	D	Y	C	N	T	E	C		E	K	E	L
		V	I		I	E	U	E	Y	M		N	F	R
			E	T	F	N	D	S	R	A	T	U	F
			D	A	N	R	E	T	E	E	L	U
C	O	U	R	A	G	E	O	U	S		V	R	L
					R	C	O			E	D
E	L	B	I	S	S	O	P	C		J			

SELF ESTEEM
Puzzle # 9

```
    S S E N M L A C I T C A R P
  E R U S A E L P O W E R F U L
  T     I N V E N T I V E   P
  H U M I L I T Y D         R
  O A C E X C I T I N G     O
  U E P O           G       D
  G   C P M E E K N E S S   U
  H   N I P       I         C
  T   H   E N O   T P       T
  F     O   D E S Y   R     I
  U       N   I S U   I     V
  L         O   F S R D     E
        A S S U R A N C E
  V A L U E           M O D E S T Y
    M O R A L E V I T C A O R P
```

SELF ESTEEM
Puzzle # 10

```
            C A P A B L E
  B R I L L I A N T
  A     S   E T N E T E P M O C
  E T   S C L S R     H
      V H   E U B I E   G
      I L   N L A U S     I
  E M O S E W A L T T R P   R
  W       I T S G L U P T E   B
  O         C I I N E R A L C
  R           E C S I W E D A T
  T             D D E R O D A
  H   A U T H E N T I C U
  Y E L B A M I T S E     S L
    C O M M E N D A B L E A L
  S U O E T R U O C             A
```

SELF ESTEEM
Puzzle # 11

```
  M E T I C U L O U S       P
      L R O T A I T I N I   O
  I N D U S T R I O U S     S
      P   F       E         I O
      R       R A   L V     T R
      E       E C   A I     I I
      C           E H R C T V G
  P   I             H I E I C E I
  A   S   B A L A N C E D G A N
  T N E D N E P E D N I V A O A
  I D I P L O M A T I C   E E L
  E           R O T A I D E M R L
  N E V I T A R E P O O C
  T       E M O T I O N A L
    O U T G O I N G
```

SELF LOVE
Puzzle # 12

```
  H E A L T H Y       D       R
  S   T T N E U Q O L E M E   A
  L U E I           J S I M   D
  L U O N S   C     O E N P   I
    O F L C I   I   V R D O   A
  G E V E U H U   M I V F W   N
  R E L I P B A Q   A I U E   T
  A   V A N O A N X L N L R G
  C     O T G H F T E G Y E L
  I     E L E C T R I C   D O
  O       V D         N     R
  U   D E R I P S N I G     I
  S J U B I L A N T D E S I O P
    T N E S E R P G         U
        L I B E R A T E D S
```

UNIQUE SELF WORTH
Puzzle # 13

```
    O   L A C I T I L O P   P
    R       D             S E
    G E V I T A N I G A M I R
P A     L U F P L E H   N S
E N P E R C E P T I V E C O
R I   E L B A I M A   S E N
S Z             M B O R A
U E       E     B   L E B
A F D   G     L   I   E L
S Y O     E S I W B T   D   E
I   T C S E N S I T I V E
V   T U     U     O X
E       I S U O I R U C E
          W E S E N S I B L E
  S K I L L E D       E       F
```

VALUES
Puzzle # 14

```
G T     G N I T S E R E T N I
  N N   E G D E L W O N K
S   I A L   N E V O L F L E S
E T   W G U K I N D N E S S
L H   I O E F   T W
F R   S   L L P   I E
A I   H A N G E L I C A
W L   F   G       E A X L
A L S U       R       H D E T
R E   L A D V E N T U R E   H
E D       A U T H E N T I C P
C I F I R R E T   A         T
    Y L T P M O R P   B
S S E C C U S M E V O L
D E T A V I T O M E A G E R
```

WHY I LOVE ME
Puzzle # 15

```
    G T N E T S I S R E P
    E L B A R O N O H N       R
    N L P A T I E N C E       E
G E   B Y T I R G E T N I     S
  R   A O T         W F       I
T O A I C N I       O A       L
R U G T N C   S     R I B R   I
U S O N I N O   O   K T I E   E
S N   P I T O U     I E H B P N
T   O   T R U V N   R F L U C
I   I   I U D A T   U I T E
N       S   M T E T A L C A
G       S   I R     I B A B
Y T I R U T A M S U   V L L
              P   M N   E E
```

WHY I LOVE ME
Puzzle # 16

```
O P P O R T U N I T Y
  P R E S T I G E R U T U F
  B R A V E Y L I M A F
    E   D B   G         B
C     A R I S T O C R A T I C
  O S   U R L Y     L       R
F H L R   T N I A   O     T F
R I   L E H Y O G D   I   H R
I S   E D   T I E I     B R E
E T       A L   R T N L   I E
N O       Y G E   E A C O G D
D R S T E S N U S   B C E H O
S Y             E     I U T M
    Y T I L I B I S S O P L D
        E R U T L U C         E
```